Total body
Reset:

Unlocking the Strategies for Sustainable Weight Control

Rose J. Wehner

Contents

Introduction
Weight Loss is Gradual

The fitness industry has undergone significant evolution, introducing various tools from food calculating scales to slimming belts. Scrolling through Instagram reveals the prevalence of weight loss diets and viral smoothie trends, often promising instant results. However, this influx of trends and advancements has added complexity to the process of losing weight. For beginners seeking weight loss or those wanting to grasp the fundamentals, this guide provides answers to frequently asked questions, simplifying the transformation process.

Contrary to the enticing promises of quick fixes and overnight transformations, weight loss is a gradual journey that demands adherence to a disciplined regimen for a minimum of six weeks to yield tangible results. While bloating can be alleviated overnight, shedding substantial weight within such a timeframe is a misconception. Beverages claiming overnight efficacy typically assist in detoxifying the body, potentially reflecting changes on the scale the next day but leaving body fat unchanged.

This book outlines procedures to be followed for achieving effective weight loss. Stay connected and read through!

Chapter 1
Impact of Weight on Health

Deciphering the body's composition is integral to comprehending the health implications of weight. The distribution of fat and muscle mass significantly shapes health outcomes, with excess adipose tissue, especially around vital organs, contributing to various health issues. Elevated fat mass is linked to an increased risk of cardiovascular diseases, diabetes, and metabolic disorders.

Weight is intricately tied to metabolic processes, where excess weight, particularly visceral fat, can disrupt hormonal balance and result in insulin resistance, a precursor to Type 2 diabetes. Additionally, adipose tissue releases inflammatory cytokines, fostering a chronic inflammatory state that exacerbates metabolic dysfunction.

The impact of weight on cardiovascular health is profound, as excess weight strains the heart, leading to conditions like hypertension and atherosclerosis. The heightened cardiovascular workload increases the risk of heart attacks and strokes. Understanding the intricate relationship between weight, blood pressure, and cholesterol levels is crucial for assessing cardiovascular health.

Weight significantly affects the musculoskeletal system, influencing joint health and overall mobility. Excess body weight stresses joints, potentially causing conditions such as osteoarthritis. Maintaining a healthy weight is vital for preserving bone density and reducing the risk of fractures and skeletal disorders.

Beyond the physiological, weight has a substantial psychological impact, intertwining with body image, self-esteem, and mental health. Understanding the psychological aspects of weight is crucial for devising holistic health management approaches. Negative body image and low self-esteem can contribute to unhealthy lifestyle choices, perpetuating a cycle of weight-related health issues.

The endocrine system, responsible for hormone regulation, is profoundly impacted by weight fluctuations. Adipose tissue acts as an endocrine organ, releasing hormones influencing appetite, metabolism, and energy balance. Dysregulation of these hormonal signals can lead to imbalances in energy homeostasis, contributing to weight gain or difficulty in losing weight.

The impact of weight on health is not uniform, with genetic and environmental factors playing pivotal roles. Genetic predispositions influence susceptibility to weight-related conditions, while environmental factors like diet, physical activity, and socio-economic status contribute to the intricate web of weight and health dynamics.

Weight plays a crucial role in reproductive health, particularly during pregnancy, where both underweight and overweight conditions can impact fertility and pose risks. Understanding weight management nuances is essential for ensuring healthy pregnancies and reducing complications for both the mother and developing fetus.

The impact of weight on health extends beyond adults, with childhood obesity emerging as a significant public health concern. Early-life weight patterns set the stage for lifelong health outcomes, with childhood obesity linked to an increased risk of chronic conditions in adulthood. Addressing weight-related issues in early life is pivotal for long-term health.

Understanding the impact of weight on health requires comprehensive interventions and management strategies. Lifestyle modifications, including dietary changes and increased physical activity, form the foundation of weight management. Behavioral interventions, such as cognitive-behavioral therapy, are crucial for addressing psychological aspects linked to weight.

For individuals with severe obesity or related health complications, medical interventions like pharmacotherapy and bariatric surgery are considerations aiming to achieve sustainable weight loss and mitigate associated health risks.

Chapter 2
Potential Health Issues Influencing Weight

Metabolic disorders, including hypothyroidism and polycystic ovary syndrome (PCOS), are pivotal health issues influencing weight. An underactive thyroid gland in hypothyroidism slows down metabolism, leading to weight gain, while PCOS, a common hormonal disorder in women, is associated with insulin resistance and weight fluctuations.

Changes in body weight can be induced by medications prescribed for various health conditions, such as corticosteroids, antidepressants, and antipsychotics. Known to be associated with weight gain, these medications require healthcare professionals to consider both the primary health issue and potential weight-related consequences in treatment planning.

Gastrointestinal disorders significantly impact weight through their effects on nutrient absorption and digestion. Conditions like celiac disease, inflammatory bowel disease (IBD), and chronic pancreatitis can result in nutrient malabsorption and weight loss. Conversely, irritable bowel syndrome (IBS) may contribute to weight fluctuations through factors like bloating and altered eating patterns.

Disruptions in hormonal levels play a crucial role in weight regulation, with imbalances in cortisol contributing to abdominal weight gain. Additionally, disturbances in sex hormone balance, such as estrogen and testosterone, may influence body composition and weight distribution.

The connection between mental health and weight is evident in psychiatric disorders like depression and anxiety, impacting appetite and eating behaviors. Severe disturbances in eating patterns characterize eating disorders such as anorexia nervosa, bulimia nervosa, and binge-eating disorder, leading to significant weight fluctuations.

Chronic inflammatory conditions like rheumatoid arthritis and systemic lupus erythematosus affect weight due to the body's inflammatory response. Increased metabolic demands and altered energy expenditure may result from inflammation, influencing weight in individuals with these conditions. Medications used for managing chronic inflammatory disorders may also have weight-related side effects.

Genetic factors significantly influence an individual's susceptibility to health conditions, contributing to weight-related challenges. Predispositions to obesity, diabetes, and cardiovascular diseases underscore the importance of understanding the genetic component for personalized approaches to weight management.

Sleep disorders, including sleep apnea and insomnia, impact weight through disruptions in hormonal regulation, leading to imbalances in ghrelin and leptin. Sleep deprivation influences food choices, contributing to overeating and weight gain.

Health issues affecting joint and mobility can influence weight by restricting physical activity. Conditions like osteoarthritis and rheumatoid arthritis may lead to a sedentary lifestyle and weight gain. Conversely, excess weight can exacerbate joint issues, creating a complex interplay between health conditions and body weight.

Reproductive health issues in women, such as PCOS, endometriosis, and hormonal imbalances, contribute to weight challenges. Hormonal changes associated with pregnancy and menopause also influence body weight and fat distribution, emphasizing the intricate relationship between reproductive health and weight.

Chapter 3
Health Benefits of Weight Loss

One of the primary advantages of weight loss lies in the enhancement of metabolic health. Excessive weight, particularly abdominal fat, is closely associated with insulin resistance, a condition where cells inadequately respond to insulin. Implementing weight loss strategies, especially through dietary changes and increased physical activity, can improve insulin sensitivity, resulting in better blood sugar control. This improvement plays a crucial role in preventing and managing Type 2 diabetes, a condition intricately connected to metabolic dysfunction.

Weight loss carries profound implications for cardiovascular health. Excess weight contributes to elevated blood pressure, atherosclerosis, and an increased risk of heart disease. Through weight loss, particularly in individuals with obesity, there is a noticeable reduction in these cardiovascular risk factors. Mechanisms involve a decrease in inflammatory markers, improved lipid profiles, and enhanced endothelial function, collectively contributing to a healthier cardiovascular system.

Adipose tissue, particularly visceral fat, functions as an endocrine organ producing inflammatory cytokines. These markers are implicated in chronic low-grade inflammation associated with obesity and various chronic diseases. Weight loss, especially through lifestyle modifications, leads to a decrease in these inflammatory markers, fostering an anti-inflammatory state within the body. This positively influences immune function, contributing to overall health and disease prevention.

Non-alcoholic fatty liver disease (NAFLD) is a common consequence of obesity, characterized by fat accumulation in the liver. Weight loss has been proven to reduce liver fat content and improve liver function. This involves a reduction in triglyceride accumulation in hepatocytes, leading to a reversal of fatty liver disease. Additionally, weight loss is associated with a decrease in liver inflammation, mitigating the progression of NAFLD.

Obesity is intricately linked to impaired respiratory function, including conditions like obstructive sleep apnea and decreased lung capacity. Weight loss contributes to improved respiratory mechanics, reducing the severity of sleep apnea and enhancing overall lung function. Mechanisms involve a reduction in inflammation in the respiratory system and decreased pressure on the airways, leading to improved respiratory efficiency.

Excess weight places additional stress on the musculoskeletal system, resulting in conditions such as osteoarthritis. Weight loss, especially in individuals with obesity, is associated with a decrease in joint pain and improved mobility. Aspects involve a reduction in the load on weight-bearing joints, leading to decreased wear and tear on cartilage and overall preservation of joint health.

Weight loss influences hormonal regulation, impacting key hormones involved in appetite control, metabolism, and energy balance. Leptin and ghrelin, known as the "hunger hormones," undergo favorable changes with weight loss. Leptin sensitivity improves, leading to enhanced satiety signals, while ghrelin levels decrease, reducing appetite. These hormonal shifts contribute to a more regulated and balanced energy intake, aiding in weight maintenance.

Obesity is often associated with sleep disturbances, including conditions like insomnia and sleep apnea. Weight loss has been shown to improve sleep quality through various mechanisms. Reductions in inflammatory markers, improvements in respiratory function, and hormonal regulation collectively contribute to better sleep patterns. The intricacies involve a complex interplay of physiological changes that positively impact the sleep-wake cycle.

Weight loss extends to cognitive benefits, influencing brain health and function. Obesity is associated with increased inflammation in the brain, contributing to cognitive decline. Weight loss, especially through lifestyle modifications, leads to a reduction in neuroinflammation and improved cognitive function. Additionally, the positive effects on insulin sensitivity and cardiovascular health contribute to enhanced brain health.

The dimensions of weight loss also extend to psychological well-being. Obesity is associated with an increased risk of depression, anxiety, and other mental health conditions. Weight loss has been shown to positively influence mood and overall psychological well-being. Mechanisms involve changes in neurotransmitter levels, including serotonin and dopamine, as well as improvements in self-esteem and body image perception.

Obesity is a recognized risk factor for certain types of cancer, including breast, colorectal, and endometrial cancers. Weight loss contributes to a reduction in cancer risk through various mechanisms. The intricacies involve a decrease in chronic inflammation, improvements in insulin sensitivity, and alterations in hormonal regulation, all of which collectively contribute to a lower risk of cancer development.

Weight loss is associated with increased longevity and a deceleration of the aging process. Obesity is linked to accelerated aging at the cellular level, including shortened telomeres and increased oxidative stress. Weight loss interventions, especially those promoting healthy lifestyle changes, have been shown to slow down these aging processes. Aspects involve a reduction in cellular damage, improvements in mitochondrial function, and enhanced cellular repair mechanisms.

Chapter 4
The Appropriate and Healthy Weight

The Body Mass Index (BMI) is a commonly employed tool for evaluating body weight, calculated by dividing an individual's weight in kilograms by the square of their height in meters. Despite its widespread use, BMI has limitations, as it doesn't consider variations in body composition, such as muscle and fat distribution. Athletes with higher muscle mass may be misclassified as overweight or obese based on BMI alone, highlighting the need for a more nuanced approach.

A more sophisticated method for weight assessment involves body composition analysis, evaluating the proportion of fat, muscle, water, and bone. Technologies like Dual-Energy X-ray Absorptiometry (DEXA), bioelectrical impedance analysis (BIA), and air displacement plethysmography provide precise insights. Analyzing fat mass and lean body mass enables tailored weight management strategies for optimized health outcomes.

Beyond overall weight, the distribution of body fat, assessed through the waist-to-hip ratio, plays a critical role in health. Accumulation of visceral fat around internal organs is linked to an increased risk of metabolic disorders and cardiovascular diseases. Even individuals with normal BMI values may have an unhealthy fat distribution pattern, emphasizing the importance of the waist-to-hip ratio.

Genetic factors significantly influence an individual's predisposition to body types and weight-related conditions, with specific genes associated with metabolism, fat storage, and appetite regulation. Understanding the genetic component aids in personalized weight management, where genetic testing contributes to a tailored approach.

Metabolic rate, especially Basal Metabolic Rate (BMR), influences the energy required for essential physiological functions. Factors such as age, gender, muscle mass, and overall health impact metabolic rate. Calculating energy needs based on metabolic rate is crucial for developing personalized nutrition plans.

Caloric balance, the equilibrium between consumed and expended calories, is fundamental to weight management. Achieving a balanced caloric equation involves considering factors like activity level, metabolic rate, and individual goals.

Macronutrient composition in the diet, including proteins, fats, and carbohydrates, plays a critical role in weight management. A diet rich in nutrient-dense foods contributes to a healthier weight, emphasizing the impact of dietary choices on metabolism and energy utilization.

Hormones like Leptin and ghrelin, known as "hunger hormones," influence appetite regulation. Imbalances in these hormones can lead to overeating and weight gain, highlighting the importance of interventions targeting hormonal regulation.

Determining an appropriate and healthy weight extends beyond physiological factors to psychosocial aspects. Emotional eating, stress-related behaviors, and cultural influences significantly impact eating habits and weight, emphasizing the need for interventions addressing these psychosocial factors.

Physical activity is essential for healthy weight management, influencing energy expenditure, muscle mass, and metabolic health. Understanding how different types of physical activity impact the body is crucial for optimizing the benefits of exercise.

Certain health conditions, such as chronic diseases, hormonal disorders, and medication-induced weight changes, complicate the determination of a healthy weight. Collaborative efforts between healthcare professionals are crucial for managing weight in the presence of underlying health conditions.

Chapter 5
Establish Weight Loss Goals

Before defining weight loss objectives, conducting a thorough analysis of body composition is vital. While traditional metrics like Body Mass Index (BMI) offer a basic overview, advanced technologies such as Dual-Energy X-ray Absorptiometry (DEXA), bioelectrical impedance analysis (BIA), and hydrostatic weighing provide precise insights into fat, muscle, and other components. This approach enables a more accurate assessment and the formulation of personalized goals.

In goal setting, understanding an individual's metabolic rate is crucial. Basal Metabolic Rate (BMR) and Total Daily Energy Expenditure (TDEE) determine appropriate caloric intake for weight loss without compromising bodily functions. Considering factors like age, gender, muscle mass, and overall health ensures personalized metabolic parameters.

Safety and sustainability are crucial considerations in setting weight loss goals. Rapid weight loss may yield initial results but risks muscle loss and metabolic health. A conservative approach, targeting 1-2 pounds per week as suggested by the American Council on Exercise, focuses on fat loss while minimizing nutrient deficiencies and muscle catabolism. Assessing individual factors guides customized weight loss rates for optimal health outcomes.

Weight loss goals should extend beyond numerical targets to broader health objectives. Considering existing health conditions, risk factors, and the impact of weight on specific health markers is crucial. For those with conditions like diabetes or cardiovascular disease, weight loss objectives may be linked to improving metabolic parameters. Aligning goals with individual health priorities is a personalized approach.

Goal setting involves understanding behavioral psychology through SMART goals. Specific, Measurable, Achievable, Relevant, and Time-bound principles ensure effective goal establishment, providing a framework for implementation.

Intricacies of goal setting include a comprehensive assessment of dietary factors. A macronutrient-focused approach considers the roles of proteins, fats, and carbohydrates in energy balance and metabolic regulation. Precision nutrition, customizing dietary plans based on individual needs, considers factors like metabolic rate and health conditions. Assessments guide the formulation of dietary goals for successful weight loss.

Acknowledging the role of physical activity, exercise physiology principles guide activity-related goals. Balancing aerobic and resistance training based on individual capabilities and a preference is crucial. Understanding energy expenditure during exercise contributes to overall goal setting.

Establishing weight loss goals is an ongoing process requiring continuous monitoring and adjustments. Regular evaluations through metrics like body composition analysis and adherence to plans allow dynamic adjustments based on individual responses.

Psychological aspects are acknowledged in goal setting, considering cognitive processes, emotional factors, and behavioral patterns. Cognitive-behavioral strategies address psychological barriers and enhance adherence by aligning goals with individual motivations.

Personalization is key in goal setting, involving collaborative efforts between individuals and healthcare professionals. Generic goals are less likely to yield sustainable results, considering individual preferences, cultural factors, and lifestyle constraints.

Periodization structures goals into specific timeframes or phases for a stepwise progression. Short-term, medium-term, and long-term goals ensure a challenging yet attainable journey.

Chapter 6
Weight Loss Time Frame

The determination of the timeframe for weight loss initiates with a thorough evaluation of metabolic factors. Metabolism, influenced by age, gender, muscle mass, and overall health, dictates the body's energy expenditure. Basal Metabolic Rate (BMR), representing energy expenditure at rest, forms the foundation for understanding metabolic needs. An analysis considers how these factors affect the caloric deficit needed for weight loss.

The core principle of weight loss centers on achieving a caloric deficit, where calories expended surpass those consumed. The timeframe for weight loss is closely tied to the magnitude of the caloric deficit, with approximately 3,500 calories equivalent to a pound of body weight. Creating a daily or weekly caloric deficit of 500 to 1,000 calories theoretically results in a weight loss of 1 to 2 pounds per week.

However, the subtleties of this estimation require attention to individual variations. Body composition, metabolic rate, and overall health impact how the body responds to a caloric deficit. A more detailed analysis may involve metabolic testing to precisely determine energy needs and optimize the caloric deficit for sustainable and healthy weight loss.

Estimating the timeframe for weight loss must also consider adaptive processes within the body. As individuals lose weight, metabolic rate may decrease, and the body may become more efficient in utilizing energy. Plateaus, where weight loss stalls despite continued efforts, are common and necessitate interventions. Adjustments to caloric intake, changes in exercise routines, and periodic reevaluations are essential components of a dynamic approach to weight loss estimation.

The considerations of estimating the timeframe for weight loss extend to precision nutrition, optimizing macronutrient composition for individual needs. Proteins, fats, and carbohydrates play distinct roles in metabolic processes, satiety, and overall health. An analysis considers the impact of macronutrient ratios on energy balance and the body's response to different dietary compositions.

For example, diets rich in protein may have a thermogenic effect, requiring more energy for digestion and metabolism. The intricacies involve tailoring macronutrient ratios to support muscle retention, enhance satiety, and promote efficient fat loss. Customizing dietary plans based on individual metabolic responses contributes to a more precise estimation of the timeframe for weight loss.

Estimating the timeframe for weight loss requires recognition of individual variability and genetic factors. Genetic predispositions influence an individual's response to dietary interventions, metabolic rate, and body composition.

Assessments may involve genetic testing to identify specific markers associated with weight loss and inform personalized strategies. Understanding how genetics interact with environmental factors contributes to a more nuanced estimation of the timeframe for achieving weight loss goals.

The estimation of the timeframe for weight loss integrates principles from behavioral psychology. Adherence to dietary and lifestyle changes is a critical determinant of success. Interventions may involve cognitive-behavioral strategies to address psychological barriers, enhance motivation, and foster sustainable habits. A more comprehensive approach considers the aspects of behavior change, understanding the role of habits, cues, and rewards in maintaining adherence over time.

Individual health status and medical considerations play a crucial role in the estimation of the timeframe for weight loss. Certain medical conditions, medications, and hormonal imbalances can influence weight loss outcomes. Assessments involve collaboration with healthcare professionals to identify and address underlying health issues that may impact the rate of weight loss. Additionally, considerations for safety and overall well-being contribute to a more responsible estimation of the timeframe.

The estimation of the timeframe for weight loss incorporates principles from exercise physiology. Physical activity contributes to energy expenditure, influences metabolic rate, and plays a role in body composition. An approach involves understanding how different types of exercise impact weight loss and body composition. Resistance training, for example, contributes to muscle retention and may influence the rate of fat loss. Integrating insights from exercise physiology allows for a more precise estimation of the timeframe for weight loss based on individualized activity plans.

Estimation of the timeframe for weight loss is most effective when it involves interdisciplinary collaboration. Healthcare professionals, including dietitians, physicians, exercise physiologists, and psychologists, bring specialized expertise to the table. Assessments from diverse perspectives contribute to a comprehensive understanding of individual needs and guide the formulation of realistic and attainable goals.

The estimation of the timeframe for weight loss is an iterative process that requires continuous monitoring and adjustments. Regular assessments, including body composition analysis, metabolic rate measurements, and adherence evaluations, provide insights into progress. Periodic adjustments to caloric intake, exercise routines, and behavioral strategies ensure that goals remain realistic and aligned with individual responses.

Chapter 7
Healthy Weight Management Strategies

Embarking on a journey towards a healthy weight entails navigating the intricate landscape of physiological, metabolic, and behavioral factors. Delving into effective strategies for healthy weight management requires a comprehensive grasp of the considerations that underlie the pursuit of balanced and optimal body weight, encompassing a multifaceted exploration of various aspects.

The initiation of healthy weight management revolves around a meticulous examination of metabolic factors. Metabolism, the body's conversion of food into energy, is pivotal for weight regulation. Essential to this is understanding Basal Metabolic Rate (BMR), representing energy expended at rest. Incorporating resistance training to optimize metabolic efficiency becomes crucial, as individuals with higher muscle mass tend to have elevated BMR.

At the core of healthy weight management lies the achievement of a balanced caloric intake. Caloric balance, the equilibrium between consumed and expended calories through BMR and physical activity, forms the foundation. A detailed inquiry involves precise caloric calculations based on individual needs, factoring in age, gender, activity level, and overall health.

Additionally, the nutrient composition of the diet emerges as a critical consideration. Balancing macronutrients – proteins, fats, and carbohydrates – becomes pivotal for metabolic health. Proteins aid muscle retention, fats provide essential fatty acids, and carbohydrates contribute to energy levels. Strategic interventions involve tailoring nutrient ratios to individual requirements, ensuring optimal metabolic function while meeting nutritional needs.

Exploration into healthy weight management strategies transcends into the realms of behavioral psychology. Cognitive strategies play a significant role in cultivating sustainable habits and achieving long-term success. Interventions, grounded in behavioral psychology, such as goal setting, self-monitoring, and cognitive restructuring, address psychological barriers and contribute to the effectiveness of weight management strategies.

The dimension of healthy weight management places emphasis on precision nutrition – a personalized approach to dietary planning. Understanding individual responses to different dietary compositions involves considering factors like metabolic rate, insulin sensitivity, and genetic predispositions. Tailoring nutritional interventions to specific needs contributes to more effective weight management, with assessments possibly including advanced tools like metabolic testing and genetic analysis.

Inquiries into healthy weight management extend into emerging strategies like intermittent fasting and time-restricted eating, influencing metabolic processes and promoting fat loss. The intricacies include understanding hormonal responses, metabolic adaptations, and individual tolerances. Incorporating these strategies necessitates precision in timing and adherence for optimizing metabolic benefits.

Healthy weight management strategies involve a profound understanding of hormonal regulation and appetite control, with Leptin and Ghrelin, known as the "hunger hormones," playing pivotal roles. Interventions aim to optimize hormonal balance through lifestyle modifications, dietary choices, and sleep hygiene, acknowledging how these hormones interact with metabolic processes for effective weight management.

The exploration of healthy weight management extends beyond physiological aspects to encompass psychosocial and environmental factors. Behavioral economics principles acknowledge the impact of social cues, environmental stimuli, and economic factors on dietary choices. Interventions may involve creating supportive environments, addressing emotional eating patterns, and fostering positive social influences to enhance the effectiveness of weight management strategies.

Inquiries about healthy weight management strategies require an examination of the intersection between weight and chronic diseases. Specific health conditions, such as diabetes, cardiovascular diseases, and metabolic disorders, demand precise strategies. Collaborative efforts with healthcare professionals ensure a comprehensive and personalized approach to weight management in the presence of chronic diseases.

Mindful eating, a cognitive awareness approach, is integral to healthy weight management. This strategy involves paying attention to the sensory experience of eating, recognizing hunger and fullness cues, and savoring each bite. Interventions may include mindfulness practices, cognitive-behavioral strategies, and cultivating a heightened awareness of eating behaviors, contributing to improved dietary choices and a sustainable approach to weight management.

The exploration of healthy weight management includes an examination of sleep quality and circadian rhythms. Disruptions in sleep patterns influence hormonal regulation, appetite control, and energy balance. Strategies involve optimizing sleep hygiene, addressing sleep disorders, and aligning eating patterns with circadian rhythms. Recognizing the intricate connections between sleep, metabolism, and weight regulation contributes to a holistic approach to healthy weight management.

Inquiries about healthy weight management strategies necessitate considerations for individuals on medications that may influence weight. Certain medications, including antidepressants, antipsychotics, and corticosteroids, are associated with weight changes. Interventions involve collaborating with healthcare providers to explore alternative medications or implementing strategies to mitigate weight-related side effects. Balancing the benefits of medication with weight management goals is a critical aspect of individualized strategies.

Chapter 8
Sustainable Approaches to Weight Loss

The pursuit of weight loss often encounters challenges, with the ultimate objective extending beyond shedding pounds to ensuring sustained results. The considerations for successful weight management encompass more than mere caloric deficits and exercise routines. A comprehensive exploration delves into the intricate physiological, metabolic, and behavioral factors, aiming to unravel dimensions of sustainable weight loss and strategies to prevent the common phenomenon of weight regain.

In sustainable weight loss, a critical consideration involves understanding the body's metabolic adaptations to changes in energy balance. As individuals adopt a calorie-restricted diet, the body adapts its energy expenditure to maintain equilibrium, potentially decreasing metabolic rate. Sustainable approaches necessitate periodic reassessments of caloric needs, dietary strategy adjustments, and incorporating periods of caloric maintenance to counter metabolic adaptations.

Precision nutrition, a tailored dietary planning approach based on individual needs, is integral to sustainable weight loss. The intricacies involve optimizing macronutrient ratios, considering the roles of proteins, fats, and carbohydrates in metabolic processes. Proteins support muscle retention, fats provide essential fatty acids, and carbohydrates contribute to energy levels. Sustainable approaches require an analysis of how different macronutrient compositions impact metabolism, appetite regulation, and overall adherence to dietary plans.

The aspects of sustainable weight loss extend into behavioral psychology, where understanding cognitive strategies is pivotal for fostering sustainable habits and preventing relapse. Interventions include cognitive-behavioral techniques addressing psychological barriers, enhancing motivation, and developing coping mechanisms. This approach recognizes the intricate interplay between thoughts, emotions, and behaviors, forming a foundation for sustained adherence to healthy lifestyle choices.

Sustainable weight loss favors gradual and progressive changes over drastic interventions, minimizing the shock to the body's systems and allowing for more seamless adaptations. Gradual reductions in caloric intake, incremental increases in physical activity, and progressive adjustments to behavioral habits form the backbone of sustained weight loss. This approach facilitates a controlled and manageable rate of weight loss, reducing the likelihood of metabolic adaptations that may impede long-term success.

Exploration of sustainable weight loss encompasses a comprehensive understanding of exercise physiology, recognizing that physical activity contributes not only to energy expenditure but also to improvements in metabolic health and body composition. Sustainable approaches involve a balance between aerobic exercise and resistance training, tailored to individual capabilities, with gradual intensity progression and variety to prevent plateaus.

The intricacies of sustainable weight loss include mindful eating, grounded in cognitive awareness of the eating experience. This approach involves paying attention to hunger and fullness cues, savoring each bite, and being present during meals. Interventions may include mindfulness practices, cognitive-behavioral strategies, and cultivating heightened awareness of eating behaviors. Sustainable weight loss benefits from understanding how mindful eating fosters healthier relationships with food, reduces emotional eating, and promotes intentional dietary choices.

Sustainable weight loss strategies delve into environmental influences and behavioral economics, recognizing that individuals make choices influenced by external cues, social norms, and economic factors. Approaches involve creating environments supporting healthy choices, addressing food accessibility, and leveraging behavioral economic strategies. This understanding acknowledges external factors' impact on decision-making, aiming to create an environment conducive to sustained healthy behaviors.

The exploration of sustainable weight loss includes an examination of sleep quality and circadian rhythms. Disruptions in sleep patterns can influence hormonal regulation, appetite control, and energy balance. Sustainable approaches involve optimizing sleep hygiene, addressing sleep disorders, and aligning eating patterns with circadian rhythms. Considerations include recognizing the intricate connections between sleep, metabolism, and weight regulation, emphasizing the importance of prioritizing quality sleep for sustained weight loss.

Preserving muscle mass is a priority in sustainable weight loss strategies. Muscle tissue contributes to overall metabolic rate, and its preservation is crucial for preventing declines in metabolism associated with weight loss. Interventions involve incorporating resistance training to stimulate muscle retention and ensuring adequate protein intake to support muscle health. Sustainable approaches prioritize strategies that mitigate muscle loss, contributing to long-term metabolic health and preventing the common pitfall of regaining lost weight.

Chapter9
Modifying Dietary Habits

Embarking on the journey to modify dietary habits necessitates an understanding of the intricate interplay between nutrition, metabolism, and individual health goals. The considerations for successful weight management extend beyond simple calorie counting, encompassing a nuanced examination of macronutrient composition, metabolic responses, and behavioral psychology. This exploration delves into the dimensions of modifying dietary habits, providing insights into how precise interventions can optimize nutritional choices for improved health outcomes.

The foundation of modifying dietary habits lies in precision nutrition, an approach involving the optimization of macronutrient composition – proteins, fats, and carbohydrates. Each macronutrient plays a unique role in metabolic processes, energy regulation, and overall health. Proteins are essential for muscle maintenance and repair, fats contribute to hormonal balance and nutrient absorption, and carbohydrates provide energy for daily activities.

A detailed analysis involves tailoring macronutrient ratios to individual needs and health goals. For instance, individuals with specific fitness objectives may benefit from higher protein intake to support muscle development. Precision nutrition considers factors such as metabolic rate, activity levels, and overall health status to formulate dietary plans aligned with individualized requirements.

Modifying dietary habits inherently involves managing caloric intake and achieving a balanced energy equation. The intricacies of caloric management include understanding basal metabolic rate (BMR), the energy required for essential physiological functions at rest. Achieving a caloric balance, where calories consumed match those expended through BMR and physical activity, is crucial for weight maintenance or modification.

Assessments may involve calculations based on individual energy needs, considering factors such as age, gender, and activity level. Precision in caloric management ensures that dietary modifications align with specific health objectives, whether it be weight loss, maintenance, or muscle gain.

Modifying dietary habits extends beyond macronutrients to include a focus on micronutrient density and nutrient timing. Micronutrients, such as vitamins and minerals, are essential for various physiological functions, including immune support, bone health, and antioxidant defense. Interventions involve selecting nutrient-dense foods providing a broad spectrum of essential micronutrients.

Nutrient timing, another consideration, involves strategically planning meals to optimize nutrient absorption and utilization. For example, consuming a balanced meal with proteins and carbohydrates after a workout supports muscle recovery and replenishes glycogen stores. The nuances of nutrient timing contribute to enhanced metabolic responses and overall nutritional efficacy.

Modifying dietary habits is not only a scientific endeavor but also a behavioral one. Behavioral psychology plays a crucial role in understanding the cognitive processes, emotional triggers, and environmental cues influencing eating behaviors. Interventions may include cognitive-behavioral strategies aimed at identifying and modifying unhealthy habits.

Habit formation, a critical aspect of behavioral psychology, involves implementing systematic changes over time to foster sustainable dietary modifications. Strategies may include setting specific, measurable, and achievable goals, employing positive reinforcement, and gradually introducing new habits. Understanding the intricacies of habit formation enhances the likelihood of long-term adherence to modified dietary patterns.

The personalized approach to modifying dietary habits recognizes the inherent variability among individuals. Personalization is a key consideration, as what works for one person may not be suitable for another. Assessments involve considering individual factors such as genetics, metabolism, and health conditions to tailor dietary modifications.

For example, individuals with specific genetic predispositions may respond differently to certain dietary patterns. Understanding these aspects allows for the customization of dietary interventions, optimizing outcomes based on individual needs and responses.

The dimensions of modifying dietary habits encompass effective dietary planning and meal preparation. Strategies involve creating well-balanced meals that meet nutritional goals, considering portion sizes, and incorporating a variety of nutrient-rich foods. Precision in meal planning ensures that dietary modifications are sustainable and provide the necessary nutrients for optimal health.

Meal preparation, a practical skill, involves cooking methods that preserve nutritional integrity and enhance digestibility. Considerations may include understanding cooking temperatures, selecting appropriate cooking oils, and minimizing nutrient loss during food processing. A strategic approach to dietary planning and meal preparation contributes to the practicality and effectiveness of modified dietary habits.

Modifying dietary habits can be more sustainable when culinary techniques and flavor optimization are considered. Interventions involve exploring cooking methods that enhance the palatability of healthy foods. For example, using herbs and spices to season dishes not only adds flavor but also provides additional health benefits.

Considerations may also involve experimenting with various cooking methods, such as grilling, roasting, or steaming, to retain nutritional value and enhance taste. The incorporation of culinary techniques aligns with the goal of making modified dietary habits enjoyable, increasing the likelihood of adherence.

In certain instances, modifying dietary habits may require considerations related to nutritional supplementation. While whole foods should be the primary source of nutrients, supplements can address specific deficiencies or support health objectives. Assessments involve identifying nutritional gaps and selecting supplements that complement modified dietary habits.

Fortification, another strategy, involves enhancing the nutrient content of foods. For example, fortifying certain foods with vitamin D or calcium can contribute to better bone health. Considerations in supplementation and fortification aim to optimize nutritional intake and support overall health.

Modifying dietary habits is an ongoing process that requires continuous monitoring and adjustments. Assessments involve tracking changes in weight, body composition, and metabolic markers to evaluate the effectiveness of dietary modifications. Periodic adjustments may be necessary to align dietary plans with evolving health goals, lifestyle changes, or metabolic responses.

Chapter 10
Suitable Physical Activities for Achieving Weight Goals

The pursuit of weight goals involves a multifaceted approach that encompasses dietary modifications, behavioral strategies, and, crucially, physical activity. Engaging in suitable physical activities is a cornerstone of achieving weight-related objectives, whether it be weight loss, muscle gain, or overall fitness improvement. This exploration delves into the intricacies of selecting and implementing appropriate physical activities to optimize outcomes in alignment with specific weight goals.

The selection of suitable physical activities begins with a comprehensive understanding of metabolic considerations. Different types of exercise impact the body's energy systems and metabolic rate in distinct ways. Aerobic exercises, such as running and cycling, primarily utilize oxygen to produce energy and are effective for calorie burning. Resistance training, on the other hand, enhances muscle mass, which contributes to increased resting metabolic rate.

Assessments of metabolic considerations involve tailoring exercise selection to align with specific weight goals. For individuals aiming for weight loss, a combination of aerobic and resistance training is often recommended to optimize both calorie expenditure and muscle development. Conversely, those focused on muscle gain may prioritize resistance training with progressive overload to stimulate hypertrophy.

Suitable physical activities must be prescribed based on individual factors to ensure safety, effectiveness, and adherence. Considerations involve evaluating factors such as age, fitness level, health status, and any pre-existing conditions. For individuals with joint issues, low-impact activities like swimming or cycling may be more suitable. Assessments may also include considerations for previous injuries, mobility limitations, or cardiovascular health.

The aspect of exercise prescription involves tailoring the frequency, intensity, duration, and type (FITT) of activities to individual needs. Assessments of fitness levels may include baseline measurements of aerobic capacity, strength, and flexibility to inform the development of a customized exercise program that aligns with weight goals.

A systematic approach to suitable physical activities incorporates the principles of periodization and progressive overload. Periodization involves structuring training programs into distinct phases to optimize adaptations and prevent plateaus. For weight goals, this strategy may involve cycles of focused activities, such as endurance training, strength training, or high-intensity interval training (HIIT).

Progressive overload is a key concept that involves gradually increasing the intensity or resistance of exercises to stimulate continued adaptations. For individuals aiming for muscle gain, this might involve progressively increasing weights or resistance. Assessments of load progression, exercise volume, and intensity ensure that suitable physical activities are continually challenging the body and promoting desired outcomes.

Achieving weight goals often involves improving cardiorespiratory fitness, which is the ability of the cardiovascular and respiratory systems to deliver oxygen to working muscles during sustained physical activity. Considerations for enhancing cardiorespiratory fitness may involve selecting suitable physical activities that elevate heart rate and challenge aerobic capacity.

Interval training, a strategy, alternates between periods of intense activity and periods of rest or lower-intensity activity. This approach can be particularly effective for weight loss goals, as it maximizes calorie burn during and after exercise. Assessments may involve determining optimal work-to-rest ratios, exercise intensities, and progression schemes for interval training.

For weight-related goals that involve muscle development or toning, resistance training is a fundamental component. The aspects of resistance training involve selecting appropriate exercises, determining optimal sets and repetitions, and progressively increasing resistance. Assessments may include evaluations of muscle imbalances, joint integrity, and biomechanics to customize resistance training programs.

Specificity in resistance training is a consideration that involves tailoring exercises to target particular muscle groups. For example, individuals with a focus on sculpting their lower body may prioritize exercises like squats, lunges, and leg presses. Expertise is required to ensure proper form, minimize injury risk, and maximize the effectiveness of resistance training for achieving weight goals.

Suitable physical activities for weight goals should also address flexibility and mobility. Considerations for flexibility training involve selecting exercises that improve the range of motion around joints. This is particularly relevant for individuals focusing on overall fitness and injury prevention. Assessments may involve identifying specific areas of tightness or limitation and implementing targeted flexibility exercises.

Mobility training, an aspect often integrated into warm-up routines, focuses on enhancing joint mobility and movement patterns. Assessments may involve identifying movement dysfunctions or imbalances that could impact the effectiveness of other physical activities. Addressing flexibility and mobility contributes to overall functional fitness and can enhance the performance of other exercises aimed at weight goals.

The inclusion of High-Intensity Interval Training (HIIT) in suitable physical activities is gaining popularity for its effectiveness in achieving various weight-related goals. HIIT involves short bursts of intense exercise followed by brief periods of rest or lower-intensity activity. The advantage of HIIT lies in its ability to induce metabolic adaptations that enhance calorie burning and improve cardiovascular health.

Assessments for incorporating HIIT involve considerations for individual fitness levels, appropriate exercise selection, and personalized work-to-rest ratios. The intensity of HIIT activates the anaerobic energy system, leading to an afterburn effect known as excess post-exercise oxygen consumption (EPOC). Expertise is required to optimize the balance between intensity and recovery, ensuring that HIIT aligns with specific weight goals.

Neuromuscular training, a consideration in suitable physical activities, focuses on enhancing the communication between the nervous system and muscles. This type of training involves exercises that challenge coordination, balance, and proprioception. Assessments may involve evaluating posture, movement patterns, and neuromuscular control to identify areas that require attention.

Functional movements, another aspect, mimic real-life activities and engage multiple muscle groups simultaneously. Considerations for incorporating functional movements include assessing the biomechanics of everyday activities and selecting exercises that enhance overall functionality. Integrating neuromuscular training and functional movements contributes to improved movement efficiency and reduced injury risk during other physical activities aimed at weight goals.

Suitable physical activities for achieving weight goals should also consider environmental factors and long-term sustainability. Assessments may involve evaluating access to facilities, time constraints, and personal preferences. Sustainable activities are those that individuals can maintain over the long term, contributing to the adherence to weight-related goals.

Considerations for sustainable activities involve creating diversified routines that prevent monotony and boredom. Assessments may include individual preferences, activity enjoyment, and the feasibility of incorporating physical activities into daily life. Sustainability is a key aspect that ensures individuals can continue engaging in suitable physical activities, supporting ongoing progress towards weight goals.

The approach to suitable physical activities includes continuous monitoring and adjustments. Regular assessments, such as fitness testing, body composition analysis, and performance evaluations, provide insights into progress. Adjustments to exercise programs may be necessary to address plateaus, prevent overtraining, or accommodate changes in fitness levels or goals.

Chapter 11
Personalized Weight Loss Program

Embarking on a weight loss journey requires more than generic advice; it necessitates a personalized approach that considers individual characteristics, metabolic factors, and health goals. A personalized weight loss program involves a detailed understanding of the aspects of nutrition, exercise physiology, and behavioral psychology. In this exploration, we delve into the intricacies of recommendations for a personalized weight loss program, emphasizing the importance of tailored strategies to optimize outcomes.

The foundation of a personalized weight loss program lies in a thorough metabolic assessment. This involves understanding the body's energy needs, with a key metric being the Basal Metabolic Rate (BMR). BMR represents the energy expended at rest and is influenced by factors such as age, gender, weight, and body composition. A systematic approach involves precise calculations to determine individual caloric requirements, ensuring that the energy deficit aligns with weight loss goals without compromising metabolic health.

A personalized weight loss program delves into precision nutrition, emphasizing the tailored distribution of macronutrients – proteins, fats, and carbohydrates. Proteins play a crucial role in muscle preservation, fats contribute to hormonal balance, and carbohydrates provide energy. Recommendations involve optimizing macronutrient ratios based on individual needs, considering factors like metabolic rate, activity level, and dietary preferences. This precision ensures that nutritional intake supports weight loss goals while meeting essential nutrient requirements.

The intricacies of a personalized weight loss program extend into the realm of behavioral psychology. Understanding cognitive strategies is pivotal for fostering sustainable habits and preventing relapse. Interventions may include cognitive-behavioral techniques aimed at identifying and modifying unhealthy habits. The focus is on addressing the root causes of behaviors related to eating, exercise, and self-image. Strategies involve goal setting, self-monitoring, and developing cognitive restructuring techniques to enhance adherence to the personalized program.

Exercise is a crucial component of a personalized weight loss program, and the considerations for individualized exercise prescription are paramount. A thorough assessment of an individual's fitness level, health status, and specific weight goals informs the selection and intensity of exercises. Expertise is required to tailor a program that combines aerobic exercises for calorie expenditure and resistance training for muscle preservation and metabolic efficiency. Personalized exercise prescription ensures that the program aligns with individual capabilities and preferences, maximizing effectiveness.

Recommendations for a personalized weight loss program involve principles of periodization and progressive overload. Periodization structures the exercise program into distinct phases to optimize adaptations and prevent plateaus. For weight loss, strategies may involve cycles of focused activities, such as endurance training, strength training, and high-intensity interval training (HIIT). Progressive overload, a key concept, entails gradually increasing the intensity or resistance of exercises to stimulate continued adaptations. Periodization and progressive overload ensure that the personalized exercise program remains challenging and effective.

A personalized weight loss program accounts for behavioral economics principles and environmental influences on dietary choices. Considerations involve recognizing the impact of external cues, social norms, and economic factors on individual decisions. The approach may include creating environments that support healthy choices, addressing food accessibility, and leveraging behavioral economic strategies such as incentivization and framing. Personalized strategies consider an individual's unique responses to environmental cues, enhancing the effectiveness of the weight loss program.

The dimension of a personalized weight loss program emphasizes continuous monitoring and data-driven adjustments. Regular assessments, including body composition analysis, metabolic rate measurements, and dietary evaluations, provide quantitative insights. Strategies involve leveraging technology, such as wearable devices and mobile applications, for real-time data. Analyzing this information allows for dynamic adjustments, ensuring that the weight loss program remains aligned with individual responses and goals.

A personalized weight loss program recognizes the role of psychosocial factors and addresses emotional eating patterns. Interventions involve assessing stress levels, emotional triggers, and coping mechanisms. Strategies may include incorporating mindfulness practices, cognitive-behavioral techniques, and stress management into the program. The approach recognizes the interconnectedness of emotional well-being and successful weight loss, fostering a holistic and sustainable approach.

The exploration of a personalized weight loss program includes an examination of sleep quality and circadian rhythms. Disruptions in sleep patterns can influence hormonal regulation, appetite control, and energy balance. Strategies involve optimizing sleep hygiene, addressing sleep disorders, and aligning eating patterns with circadian rhythms. Recognizing the intricate connections between sleep, metabolism, and weight regulation contributes to a holistic approach to personalized weight loss.

A personalized weight loss program acknowledges the importance of individualized support and accountability. Considerations involve assessing an individual's preferences for support mechanisms, whether through one-on-one counseling, group sessions, or digital platforms. Strategies may include regular check-ins, goal reviews, and addressing any challenges or barriers faced by the individual. Personalized support enhances motivation, adherence, and overall success in achieving weight loss goals.

For individuals with underlying health conditions, a personalized weight loss program requires collaboration with healthcare professionals. Assessments involve monitoring health parameters, such as blood pressure, cholesterol levels, and blood glucose. Strategies may include adjustments to the weight loss program based on medical considerations and collaboration with healthcare providers to ensure the safety and effectiveness of the program. A personalized approach involves tailoring strategies to accommodate specific health needs and optimize overall well-being.

Final Words

The landscape of weight loss is intricate and dynamic, requiring the understanding of individual factors, metabolic dynamics, and behavioral psychology. Precision nutrition, metabolic considerations, behavioral interventions, and environmental influences collectively shape a framework for successful weight loss. As individuals embark on this journey, the synthesis of these elements fosters an approach that is not only effective in achieving weight loss goals but is also sustainable, promoting long-term health and well-being.